CW00502352

The Complete Keto Breakfast Cookbook for Women

Amazing Breakfast Recipes to Start Your Keto Diet and Stay Fit

Britt Leonard

© Copyright 2020 - All rights reserved.

The content contained within this book may not be reproduced, duplicated or transmitted without direct written permission from the author or the publisher.

Under no circumstances will any blame or legal responsibility be held against the publisher, or author, for any damages, reparation, or monetary loss due to the information contained within this book. Either directly or indirectly.

Legal Notice:

This book is copyright protected. This book is only for personal use. You cannot amend, distribute, sell, use, quote or paraphrase any part, or the content within this book, without the consent of the author or publisher.

Disclaimer Notice:

Please note the information contained within this document is for educational and entertainment purposes only. All effort has been executed to present accurate, up to date, and reliable, complete information. No warranties of any kind are declared or implied. Readers acknowledge that the author is not engaging in the rendering of legal, financial, medical or professional advice. The content within this book has been derived from various sources. Please consult a licensed professional before attempting any techniques outlined in this book.

By reading this document, the reader agrees that under no circumstances is the author responsible for any losses, direct or indirect, which are incurred as a result of the use of information contained within this document, including, but not limited to, — errors, omissions, or inaccuracies.

Table of contents

Pumpkin Bread and Salmon Sandwich...............................5

Low-Carb Pancakes with Cream and Raspberries...........9

Spicy Eggs with Cheese...11

Scrambled Eggs with Salmon.......................................13

Vinaigrette And Mushroom Frittata..............................15

Shrimp And Chives Omelet...18

Goat Cheese And Asparagus Omelet.............................21

Creamy Bagel Omelet..24

Cheesy Bacon Egg Cups..26

Buttery Eggs with Avocado and Spinach.......................28

Spicy Cheesy Eggs with Avocado and Cilantro..............30

Keto Kale and Bacon with Eggs...................................33

Keto Cereal...35

Crunchy Cinnamon French Toast.................................38

Coffee Chia Smoothie..41

Everything Bagel Seasoned Eggs.................................43

Beef & Veggie Hash..45

Eggs & Spinach Florentine..47

Walnut Granola...49

Creamy Bacon Omelet...51

Sausage Breakfast..53

Chicken And Egg Stuffed Avocado...............................55

Bacon And Broccoli Egg Muffins..................................57

Scrambled Eggs with Cheese and Chili.........................59

Stevia Chocolate Waffle..61

Almond Cream Cheese Pancakes... 63

Simple Scrambled Eggs.. 65

Basic Capicola Egg Cups.. 67

Easy Sausage, Egg, And Cheese Casserole........................ 69

Waffle Sandwiches... 71

Lemon Allspice Muffins.. 74

Keto Cinnamon Flaxseed Bun Muffins................................ 76

Bacon Quiche... 78

Low Carb Jambalaya with Chicken...................................... 81

Sausage And Spinach Hash Bowl.. 83

Healthy Hemp Seed Porridge.. 85

Nut-Free Granola with Clusters.. 87

Creamy Spanish Scrambled Eggs.. 90

Spanish Egg Frittata.. 92

Basic Cream Crepes.. 94

Strawberry Smoothie Bowl.. 96

Breadless Egg Sandwich... 98

Ham And Veggie Omelet in A Bag...................................... 100

Classic Omelet... 102

Paleo Omelet Muffins... 104

Easy Enchilada Chicken Dip... 106

Grilled Portobello Mushrooms.. 108

Pumpkin Bread and Salmon Sandwich

Macros: Fat 80% | Protein 17% | Carbs 3%

Prep time: 5 minutes | Cook time: 1 hour 10 minutes | Serves 2

It is a keto sandwich that is perfect for brunch with fellow friends. It can be a holiday breakfast, too. It is simple to prepare the meal. The salmon sandwich never fails to impress.

SPICY PUMPKIN BREAD:

1 tablespoon melted coconut oil, for greasing the pan

2 tablespoons pumpkin pie spice

1 teaspoon salt

⅓ cup chopped walnuts

⅓ cup pumpkin seeds, plus more for topping

1¼ cups coconut flour

2 tablespoons ground psyllium husk powder

1¼ cups almond flour

1 tablespoon baking powder

½ cup flaxseed

3 eggs

14 ounces (397 g) pumpkin purée

¼ cup melted coconut oil

½ cup unsweetened apple sauce

TOPPINGS:

2 tablespoons heavy whipping cream

4 eggs

Salt and freshly ground black pepper, to taste

2 ounces (57 g) butter, for frying

1 pinch chili flakes

2 tablespoons melted butter

1 ounce (28 g) leafy lettuce greens

3 ounces (85 g) smoked salmon

1 tablespoon chopped fresh chives

MAKE THE SPICY PUMPKIN BREAD:

1. Preheat the oven to 400°F (205°C). Grease a bread pan with melted coconut oil and set aside.

2. In a bowl, add pumpkin pie spice, salt, walnuts, pumpkin seeds, coconut flour, husk powder, almond flour, baking powder, and flaxseed and mix.

3. In a separate bowl, whisk together eggs, pumpkin purée, oil and apple sauce until smooth. Add the dry ingredients to the bowl of wet ingredients. Stir well with a fork until it forms a smooth batter.

4. Pour the batter into the greased baking dish and smooth the top with a spatula. Scatter the top with a tablespoon of pumpkin seeds.

5. Bake in the preheated oven for 1 hour or until a toothpick inserted in the center comes out clean.

6. Allow to cool for 8 minutes before slicing and set aside.

MAKE THE SANDWICH:

7. In a bowl, add the cream and eggs and whisk to combine. Sprinkle pepper and salt to season.

8. In a frying pan, add the butter and melt over medium high heat. Add the egg mixture and cook for about 4 minutes until scrambled, stirring occasionally. Remove from the heat to a plate, then sprinkle with chili flakes. Set aside.

9. Lay the pumpkin bread slices on a clean work surface and brush with melted butter.

10. Top with scrambled eggs, lettuce leaves, salmon and chopped chives, then serve.

STORAGE: Store in an airtight container in the fridge for up to 4 days. It is not recommended to freeze.

REHEAT: Microwave, covered, until the desired temperature is reached or reheat in a frying pan or air fryer / instant pot, covered, on medium.

SERVE IT WITH: To make this a complete meal, serve the dish with a cup of strawberry avocado smoothie.

PER SERVING

calories: 571 | fat: 51.0g | total carbs: 10.0g | fiber: 6.0g | protein: 24.0g

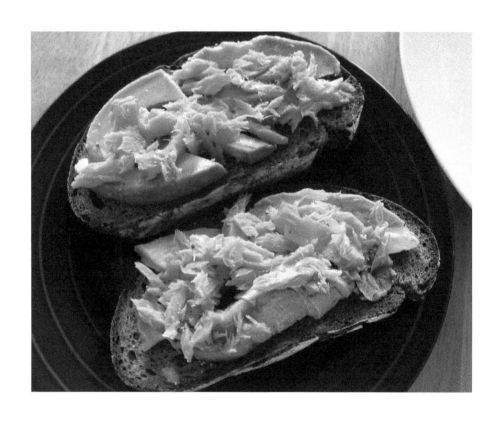

Low-Carb Pancakes with Cream and Raspberries

Macros: Fat 84% | Protein 13% | Carbs 3%

Prep time: 5 minutes | Cook time: 5 minutes | Serves 4

T hese are delicious keto pancakes. When you try this pancake, you will never look back to the ordinary pancakes. The berry topping gives it the sweetness and flavor. You should definitely try out this recipe.

PANCAKES:

4 eggs

1 tablespoon ground psyllium husk powder

7 ounces (198 g) cottage cheese

2 ounces (57 g) coconut oil

TOPPINGS:

1 cup heavy whipping cream

2 ounces (57 g) fresh raspberries

1. Whisk the eggs in a bowl and add psyllium husk and cottage cheese. Stir to combine until you get a smooth batter.

2. In a large skillet, melt the coconut oil over medium heat.

3. Pour the batter into the skillet and tilt the pan so it spreads all over. Cook for about 2 to 3 minutes until

golden brown. Carefully flip it over and cook for 1 minute more.

4. Transfer the pancake to a plate. Serve topped with heavy cream and raspberries.

STORAGE: Store in an airtight container in the fridge for up to 4 days. It is not recommended to freeze.

REHEAT: Microwave the pancakes, covered, until the desired temperature is reached or reheat in a frying pan or air fryer / instant pot, covered, on medium.

SERVE IT WITH: To make this a complete meal, serve the dish with a cup of green keto smoothie.

PER SERVING

calories: 428 | fat: 40.0g | total carbs: 7.0g | fiber: 4.0g | protein: 14.0g

Spicy Eggs with Cheese

Macros: Fat 73% | Protein 24% | Carbs 3%

Prep time: 5 minutes | Cook time: 10 minutes | Serves 1

It is an easy to prepare low-carb and keto-friendly breakfast. One can take it as lunch or dinner. The oregano spicing up the color and flavor sums up the deliciousness of the meal.

½ tomato

Salt and freshly ground black pepper, to taste

½ tablespoon butter

2 eggs

2 ounces (57 g) cubed Cheddar cheese

½ teaspoon dried oregano

1. In a bowl, season the tomato with salt and pepper.

2. Melt the butter in a frying pan over medium heat. Add the tomato, cut side down, and break the eggs into the pan.

3. Fry them for about 4 minutes, flipping the eggs and tomato halfway through the cooking time, or until cooked to your desired doneness. Season with salt and pepper.

4. Transfer the eggs to a serving plate. Top with fried tomato, cheese and oregano before serving.

STORAGE: Store in an airtight container in the fridge for up to 4 days. It is not recommended to freeze.

REHEAT: Microwave the eggs and tomato, covered, until the desired temperature is reached or reheat in a frying pan or air fryer / instant pot, covered, on medium.

SERVE IT WITH: To make this a complete meal, serve with sugar-free chocolate butter smoothie.

PER SERVING

calories: 396 | fat: 32.0g | total carbs: 5.0g | fiber: 2.0g | protein: 24.0g

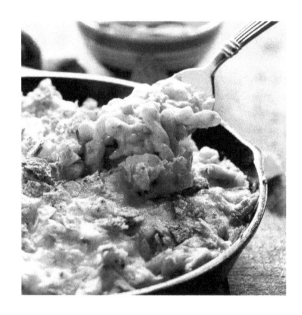

Scrambled Eggs with Salmon

Macros: Fat 73% | Protein 25% | Carbs 2%

Prep time: 2 minutes | Cook time: 10 minutes | Serves 1

T he meal takes less time as it is simple to prepare and cook. The meal is rich in nutrients and flavors. Addition of the chives and pepper adds flavor and taste to the food.

2 eggs, whisked

2 tablespoons butter

¼ cup heavy whipping cream

1 tablespoon chopped fresh chives

Salt and freshly ground black pepper, to taste

2 ounces (57 g) cured salmon

1. In a frying pan, add butter and heat until it melts. Pour the eggs and cream into the pan and stir until scrambled.
2. Lower the heat and allow the mixture to simmer for a few minutes. Continue stirring the mixture until creamy. Sprinkle with the chives, pepper, and salt.
3. Transfer the egg mixture to a platter and serve with cured salmon on the side.

STORAGE: Store in an airtight container in the fridge for up to 4 days. It is not recommended to freeze.

REHEAT: Microwave, covered, until the desired temperature is reached or reheat in a frying pan or air fryer / instant pot, covered, on medium.

SERVE IT WITH: To make this a complete meal, serve with lemon cucumber smoothie.

PER SERVING

calories: 749 | fat: 61.0g | total carbs: 3.0g | fiber: 0g | protein: 47.0g

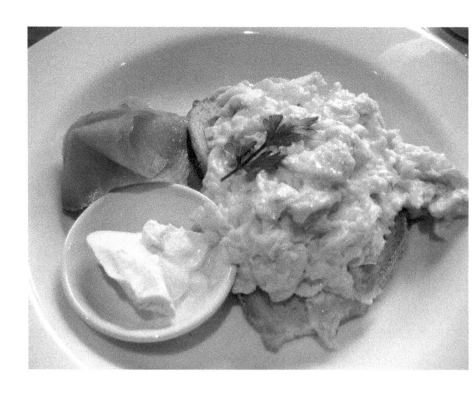

Vinaigrette And Mushroom Frittata
Macros: Fat 86% | Protein 12% | Carbs 2%

Prep time: 15 minutes | Cook time: 40 minutes | Serves 4

T his recipe is versatile as you can take during any meal session. And it is also easy to prepare. Famously referred to as the Italy's open-faced omelet. It is a keto classic meal with the excellent complement to the eggs.

VINAIGRETTE:

4 tablespoons olive oil

1 tablespoon white wine vinegar

FRITTATA:

1 pound (454 g) sliced mushrooms

4 ounces (113 g) butter

6 chopped scallions

1 teaspoon salt

½ teaspoon ground black pepper

1 tablespoon fresh parsley

10 eggs

8 ounces (227 g) shredded cheese

1 cup keto-friendly mayonnaise

½ teaspoon salt

¼ teaspoon ground black pepper

4 ounces (113 g) leafy greens

1. Preheat the oven to 350°F (180°C).
2. Make the vinaigrette: In a bowl, combine the olive oil and vinegar. Stir well to combine. Set aside.
3. Make the frittata: Melt the butter in a nonstick skillet over medium-high heat, then add and sauté the mushrooms until lightly browned. Remove from the heat and reserve the melted butter to grease a baking dish.
4. On a plate, combine the scallions with fried mushrooms, then sprinkle with salt and pepper. Fold in the parsley.
5. In another bowl, whisk together the eggs, cheese, mayonnaise, salt and pepper.
6. Add the mushroom mixture to the egg mixture. Stir to combine well.
7. Pour the mixture into the greased baking dish. Arrange the dish in the preheated oven and bake for about 40 minutes until lightly browned and puffed.
8. Transfer to four serving plates. Allow to cool for 5 minutes, then serve with the vinaigrette and leafy greens.

STORAGE: Store in an airtight container in the fridge for up to 4 days or in the freezer for up to 1 month.

REHEAT: Microwave, covered, until the desired temperature is reached or reheat in a frying pan or air fryer / instant pot, covered, on medium.

SERVE IT WITH: To make this a complete meal, serve with keto vanilla milkshake.

PER SERVING

calories: 1084 | fat: 104.0g | total carbs: 8.0g | fiber: 3.0g | protein: 32.0g

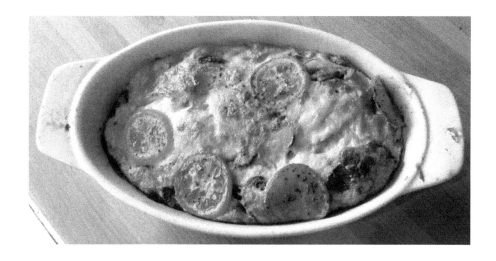

Shrimp And Chives Omelet

Macros: Fat 86% | Protein 13% | Carbs 1%

Prep time: 5 minutes | Cook time: 15 minutes | Serves 2

I t is a keto meal that is delicious and only takes 15 minutes to cook. The folds of the omelet bring together the flavors in the recipe. The dressings are simple to prepare. Why not try it today?

FILLING:

4 tablespoons olive oil, divided

5 ounces (142 g) cooked shrimp, shelled and deveined

1 red chili pepper

2 garlic cloves, minced

½ teaspoon fennel seeds

Salt and freshly ground black pepper, to taste

½ teaspoon ground cumin

1 tablespoon fresh chives

½ cup keto-friendly mayonnaise

OMELET:

6 eggs

Salt and freshly ground black pepper, to taste

1. Heat 2 tablespoons olive oil in a skillet until it shimmers.

2. Add the shrimp, chili pepper, minced garlic, fennel seeds, pepper, salt, and cumin to the skillet, then cook for 3 to 4 minutes. Transfer the mixture to a bowl to cool.
3. Add the chives and mayonnaise to the mixture. Stir to combine well and set aside.
4. In a bowl, whisk all the eggs, then sprinkle salt and pepper to season.
5. Make the omelet: In a large skillet, heat the remaining olive oil. Pour the eggs to the skillet, tilting the pan to spread it evenly. Cook for 1 to 2 minutes or until the bottom is set.
6. Pour the shrimp mixture over the omelet. Using a spatula, gently fold the omelet in half to enclose the filling. Reduce the heat, then allow the omelet to set completely.
7. Divide the omelet between two plates and serve while warm.

STORAGE: Store in an airtight container in the fridge for up to 4 days. It is not recommended to freeze.

REHEAT: Microwave, covered, until the desired temperature is reached or reheat in a frying pan or air fryer / instant pot, covered, on medium.

SERVE IT WITH: To make this a complete meal, serve the omelet with veggie salad.

PER SERVING

calories: 880 | fat: 84.0g | total carbs: 5.0g | fiber: 2.0g | protein: 28.0g

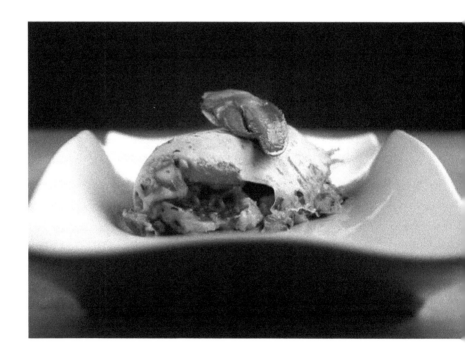

Goat Cheese And Asparagus Omelet

Macros: Fat 74% | Protein 22% | Carbs 4%

Prep time: 10 minutes | Cook time: 15 minutes | Serves 2

With fresh spring vegetables, the omelet is a pleasant choice in every energetic breakfast. The meal is full of flavor and the simplicity in making it tops it all. The meal is versatile as you can take it with almost every other meal.

4 large eggs

2 tablespoons heavy whipping cream

1 tablespoon butter

4 chopped green asparagus, cut into 1-inch pieces

Salt and freshly ground black pepper, to taste

2 ounces (57 g) goat cheese, shredded

1 ounce (28 g) baby spinach

½ chopped scallion

1. Whisk all the eggs in a bowl, then add the cream. Mix well until foamy, then set the mixture aside.

2. Melt the butter in a skillet over medium heat. Add the asparagus and sauté for approximately 4 minutes until fork-tender.

3. Transfer the asparagus to a plate and leave the melted butter in the skillet.

4. Make the omelet: Lower the heat, then pour the egg mixture into the skillet. Tilt the pan so the mixture covers the bottom of the skillet evenly. Cook for 1 minute and sprinkle with salt and pepper in the last 30 seconds. Top the omelet with cheese, asparagus and spinach on the omelet. Flip the omelet, then let it cook for 2 minutes more.
5. Divide and transfer to two serving plates. Top with the scallion and allow to cool for 5 minutes before serving.

STORAGE: Store in an airtight container in the fridge for up to 4 days. It is not recommended to freeze.

REHEAT: Microwave, covered, until the desired temperature is reached or reheat in a frying pan or air fryer / instant pot, covered, on medium.

SERVE IT WITH: To make this a complete meal, serve with turmeric keto smoothie.

PER SERVING

calories: 327 | fat: 27.0g | total carbs: 5.0g | fiber: 2.0g | protein: 18.0g

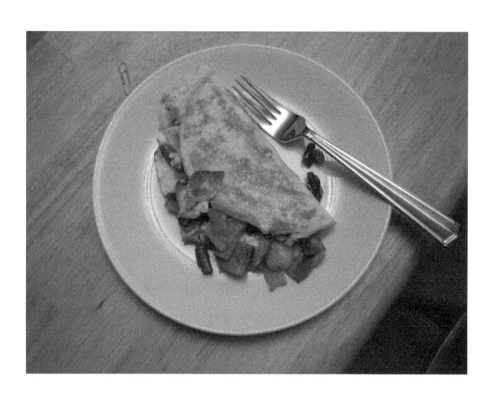

Creamy Bagel Omelet

Macros: Fat: 71% | Protein: 28% | Carbs: 1%

Prep time: 5 minutes | Cook time: 10 minutes | Serves 1

o you want to make a quick and easy breakfast? Look no further than this bagel omelet dish. Guaranteed to taste delicious, it is perfect for kids and adults alike. It is the perfect recipe for all your busy weekdays.

3 large eggs

1 tablespoon heavy whipping cream or coconut cream

1 tablespoon butter

2 ounces (57 g) smoked salmon

1 tablespoon fresh dill, minced

1 shaved scallion, divided

1 teaspoon bagel seasoning

1. Heat a medium frying pan over medium heat until it warms.

2. Whisk the eggs and whipping cream in a small bowl.

3. Put the butter in the pan, when the butter melts, tilt the pan so it covers the bottom evenly. Pour in the egg mixture and spread it all over the pan.

4. Use a spatula to mix the eggs, making sure not to scramble them.

5. Turn off the heat, then put the smoked salmon, dill, and ¾ of the scallions in the middle of the egg, then use the spatula to lift one edge of the egg to cover the filling. Roll it over until it is shaped like a tube.
6. Serve the omelet on a plate garnished with the bagel seasoning and the remaining scallions.

STORAGE: Store in an airtight container in the fridge for up to 4 days. It is not recommended to freeze.

REHEAT: Microwave, covered, until the desired temperature is reached or reheat in a frying pan or air fryer / instant pot, covered, on medium.

SERVE IT WITH: To make this a complete meal, serve it with some berries and a cup of coffee.

PER SERVING

calories: 391 | fat: 31.0g | total carbs: 1.0g | fiber: 0g | protein: 27.0g

Cheesy Bacon Egg Cups

Macros: Fat: 58% | Protein: 39% | Carbs: 3%

Prep time: 5 minutes | Cook time: 15 minutes | Serves 3

T his cheesy bacon egg cup dish is perfect for any busy weekday. Loved by kids and adults, kick things up a notch with this delicious variation of the standard breakfast recipe and you won't regret it.

3 ounces (85 g) bacon, in slices

3 ounces (85 g) Cheddar cheese, shredded

6 large eggs

Salt and freshly ground black pepper, to taste

Thinly sliced fresh basil, for garnish

SPECIAL EQUIPMENT:

A 6-cup muffin tin, lightly greased with coconut oil

1. Start by preheating the oven to 400°F (205°C).

2. Put a bacon slice in each muffin cup, making sure it curves around the well to form a bowl. Add 2 tablespoons of cheese into every bacon cup.

3. Break an egg into each cup and sprinkle with salt and pepper.

4. Put the muffin cups in the oven and bake for 12 to 14 minutes until the egg whites are set.

5. Serve hot garnished with basil.

STORAGE: Store in an airtight container in the fridge for up to 4 days or in the freezer for up to 1 month.

REHEAT: Microwave, covered, until the desired temperature is reached or reheat in an air fryer or instant pot, covered, on medium.

SERVE IT WITH: To make this a complete meal, serve it with a cup of black tea.

PER SERVING

calories: 154 | fat: 10.0g | total carbs: 1.0g | fiber: 0g | protein: 15.0g

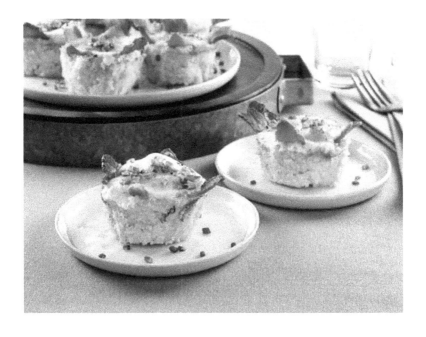

Buttery Eggs with Avocado and Spinach

Macros: Fat: 84% | Protein: 12% | Carbs: 4%

Prep time: 5 minutes | Cook time: 7 minutes | Serves 1

Looking for a light egg breakfast? Look no further than this buttery egg with avocado and spinach dish. Get those important greens in every bite with this egg recipe. It is perfect for adults with busy weekdays and for kids.

½ ounce (14 g) butter

2 eggs

Salt and freshly ground black pepper, to taste

½ avocado, scooped out and cut into wedges

1 (3-ounce / 85-g) tomato, sliced

½ cup baby spinach

1. Melt the butter in a frying pan over medium heat.
2. Break the eggs into the pan and let it fry on one side for 2 minutes for sunny-side-up eggs. For well-cooked eggs, fry for 1 minute on each side. Season with salt and pepper.
3. Transfer the fried eggs to a plate. Serve topped with avocado wedges, sliced tomatoes, and baby spinach.

STORAGE: Store in an airtight container in the fridge for up to 4 days. It is not recommended to freeze.

REHEAT: Microwave the eggs, covered, until the desired temperature is reached or reheat in a frying pan or air fryer / instant pot, covered, on medium.

SERVE IT WITH: To make this a complete meal, serve it with a cup of coffee with some cream.

PER SERVING

calories: 481 | fat: 45.0g | total carbs: 12.0g | fiber: 7.0g | protein: 14.0g

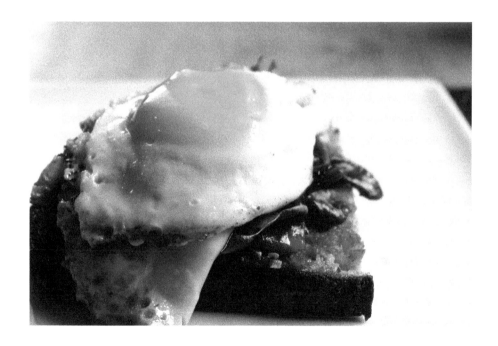

Spicy Cheesy Eggs with Avocado and Cilantro

Macros: Fat: 79% | Protein: 12% | Carbs: 9%

Prep time: 15 minutes | Cook time: 20 minutes | Serves 4

Only for the spiciest of them all, this dish is the perfect blend of cheesy deliciousness and healthy low-carb ingredients. Perfect for adults and kids who love taking bites on the wild side. The cheesy eggs dish will be your favorite.

½ cup olive oil, divided

2 fresh jalapeños, minced

1 white onion, minced

2 garlic cloves, minced

2 cups crushed tomatoes

Salt and freshly ground black pepper, to taste

8 eggs

TOPPINGS:

1 avocado, sliced

2 ounces (57 g) shredded queso fresco

4 tablespoons fresh cilantro, chopped

1. Pour ⅓ of the olive oil into a large skillet over medium heat, then add the jalapeños to cook until slightly

tender. Mix in the onions and garlic and keep stirring until the onions become translucent.

2. Pour the crushed tomatoes into the pan and reduce the heat. Let it cook until the sauce has thickened, then season with salt and pepper. Remove the tomato mixture from the heat to a plate. Set aside.

3. Pour the remaining oil into the skillet over medium heat.

4. One at a time, crack the eggs into the skillet. Fry for 2 minutes or until the egg white has set but the yolk is still runny. Sprinkle with salt and pepper. Stir in the tomato mixture and cook for 1 minute more.

5. Divide the egg mixture among four plates. Top each plate evenly with sliced avocado, queso fresco, and cilantro. Serve warm.

STORAGE: Store in an airtight container in the fridge for up to 4 days. It is not recommended to freeze.

REHEAT: Microwave the egg mixture, covered, until the desired temperature is reached or reheat in a frying pan or air fryer / instant pot, covered, on medium.

SERVE IT WITH: To make this a complete meal, serve it with a glass of sparkling water.

PER SERVING

calories: 513 | fat: 45.0g | total carbs: 17.0g | fiber: 6.0g | protein: 16.0g

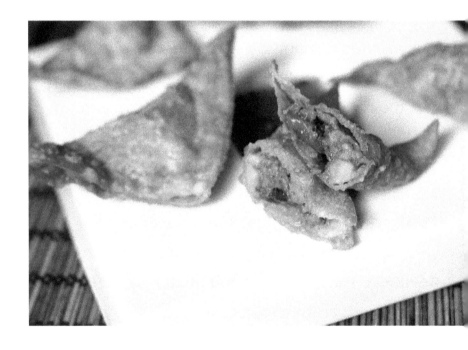

Keto Kale and Bacon with Eggs
Macros: Fat: 68% | Protein: 22% | Carbs: 10%

Prep time: 5 minutes | Cook time: 20 minutes | Serves 2

N eed to stock up on healthy and nutritious veggies? Or you just don't want to eat your veggies without some meat. This is the best combination of vegetables and other healthy food sources. This delicious dish is perfect for adults and kids.

4 ounces (113 g) bacon, chopped into bite-sized pieces

¾ pound (340 g) kale, chopped

2 eggs

Salt and freshly ground black pepper, to taste

1. Put the bacon in a large frying pan over medium heat. Cook for 4 minutes on each side or until it is crispy. Remove from the pan to a bowl and set aside.

2. Put the kale in the pan and sprinkle salt and pepper, and then cook for 2 minutes. Remove from the pan to two plates and set aside.

3. Break the eggs straight into the pan and cook for 2 minutes or until the egg white has set but the yolk is still runny. Season with salt and pepper.

4. Top each plate of kale with bacon and fried egg, then serve.

STORAGE: Store in an airtight container in the fridge for up to 4 days. It is not recommended to freeze.

REHEAT: Microwave, covered, until the desired temperature is reached or reheat in a frying pan or air fryer / instant pot, covered, on medium.

SERVE IT WITH: To make this a complete meal, serve it with a glass of sparkling water.

PER SERVING

calories: 355 | fat: 27.0g | total carbs: 14.0g | fiber: 5.0g | protein: 19.0g

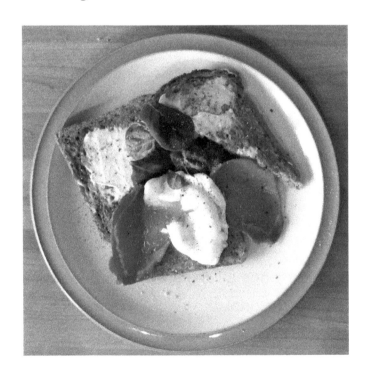

Keto Cereal

Macros: Fat: 85% | Protein: 11% | Carbs: 4%

Prep time: 15 minutes | Cook time: 15 minutes | Serves 6

H ave you finally gotten tired of walking around your supermarket or grocery store and seeing only sugar-filled cereal? Look no further than this low-carb alternative that is suitable for adults and kids. Say hello to this delicious cereal that is packed with only nutritious goodness for you and your family.

1 tablespoon golden flaxmeal

1 teaspoon ground cinnamon

1 cup almond flour

2 tablespoons sunflower seeds

1 teaspoon vanilla extract

¼ teaspoon salt

2 tablespoons water

1 tablespoon coconut oil

TO SERVE:

6 cups unsweetened almond milk

1. Start by preheating the oven to 350°F (180°C).

2. Pour the golden flaxmeal, cinnamon, flour, sunflower seeds, vanilla extract, and salt into a food processor and process until the mixture is smooth.

3. Add the water and the coconut oil to the food processor and pulse until a dough is formed.
4. Transfer the dough to a parchment paper on a flat work surface, then press until it is flat. Cover the dough with another parchment paper and roll the dough until it is 1.5 to 3 mm thick.
5. Remove the top parchment paper and cut the dough into 1-inch squares with a pizza cutter or knife.
6. Arrange the squares with the bottom layer of parchment paper on a baking sheet. Bake for 10 to 15 minutes until the edges are golden brown and crispy.
7. Let cool for 5 minutes, then serve it with unsweetened almond milk.

STORAGE: Store in an airtight container in the fridge for up to 4 days or in the freezer for up to 1 month.

REHEAT: Microwave, covered, until the desired temperature is reached or reheat in an air fryer or instant pot, covered, on medium.

SERVE IT WITH: To make this a complete meal, serve it with a glass of sparkling water.

PER SERVING

calories: 181 | fat: 17.0g | total carbs: 2.0g | fiber: 0g | protein: 5.0g

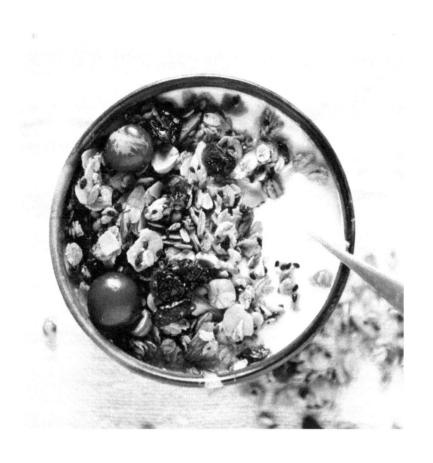

Crunchy Cinnamon French Toast

Macros: Fat: 83% | Protein: 14% | Carbs: 3%

Prep time: 5 minutes | Cook time: 15 minutes | Serves 2

French toast has never tasted better. This low-carb alternative is perfect for busy weekdays. It is very delicious and is perfect for breakfast or brunch.

MUG BREAD:

1 teaspoon melted butter

1½ teaspoons baking powder

1 pinch salt

2 tablespoons almond flour

2 tablespoons coconut flour

2 eggs, beaten

2 tablespoons heavy whipping cream

BATTER:

2 eggs

2 tablespoons heavy whipping cream

½ teaspoon ground cinnamon

1 pinch salt

2 tablespoons butter

1. Preheat the oven to 350ºF (180ºC). Grease a glass dish with melted butter and set aside.

2. In a bowl, mix the baking powder, salt, almond flour, and coconut flour with a spoon, then add the eggs and the whipping cream. Stir well until it is smooth.

3. Pour the mixture into the greased dish then put it in the microwave to cook on high pressure for 2 minutes or until a knife inserted in the middle comes out clean.

4. Remove the bread from the microwave and let cool. Slice the bread in half and set aside.

5. Mix the batter ingredients together in a bowl. Soak the bread in the bowl to coat well.

6. Arrange the bread in a baking dish and put in the oven to toast for 5 minutes on each side until golden brown.

7. Remove the bread from the oven. Let rest for 5 minutes before serving.

STORAGE: Store in an airtight container in the fridge for up to 4 days. It is not recommended to freeze.

REHEAT: Microwave, covered, until it reaches the desired temperature.

SERVE IT WITH: To make this a complete meal, serve it with a cup of green tea.

PER SERVING

calories: 392 | fat: 36.0g | total carbs: 6.0g | fiber: 3.0g | protein: 14.0g

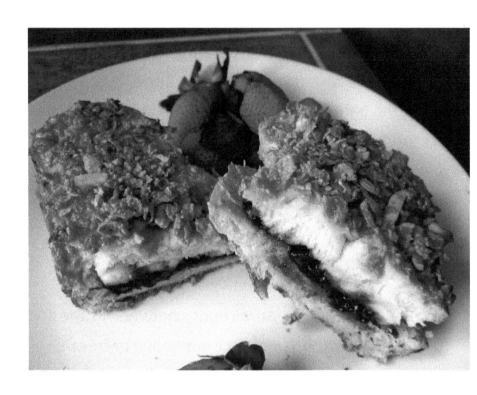

Coffee Chia Smoothie
Macros: Fat: 92% | Protein: 6% | Carbs: 2%

Prep time: 5 minutes | Cook time: 0 minutes | Serves 2

A smoothie with health benefits of coffee, chia seeds, flaxseed meal, coconut oil, almond, coconut milk compliments coffee and seeds will bring you a pleasant morning or add a soft flavor for your dinner.

2 cups unsweetened strong-brewed coffee, frozen in cubes

1 cup unsweetened almond milk

1 cup unsweetened coconut milk

2 tablespoons coconut oil

2 tablespoons chia seeds

2 tablespoons flaxseed meal

1 to 2 tablespoons granulated monk fruit sweetener

⅛ teaspoon ground cinnamon

1. Add all ingredients in a high-power blender and pulse until creamy and smooth.

2. Pour the smoothie into two glasses and serve immediately.

STORAGE: Store brewed coffee in ice cube trays and freeze for 1 to 2 weeks.

SERVE IT WITH: Serve this smoothie with the topping of heavy cream.

PER SERVING

calories: 430 | fat: 44.2g | total carbs: 6.6g | fiber: 4.5g | protein: 6.0g

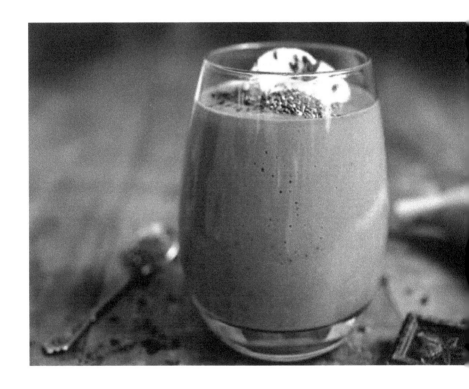

Everything Bagel Seasoned Eggs

Macros: Fat: 67% | Protein: 26% | Carbs: 7%

Prep time: 10 minutes | Cook time: 5 minutes | Serves 2

One of the simplest and easiest breakfast of boiled eggs! Spice mixture gives a deliciously spicy kick to boiled eggs.

4 eggs

3 tablespoons white sesame seeds

1 tablespoon black sesame seeds

2 teaspoons poppy seeds

1 tablespoon onion flakes

1 teaspoon garlic flakes

1 teaspoon coarse sea salt

1. In a medium saucepan of water, place the eggs over medium-high heat and bring to a boil. Boil for about 1 minute. Cover the saucepan and immediately remove from the heat. Set the pan aside, covered for about 10 minutes. Drain the eggs and transfer the eggs into a bowl of cold water to cool completely.

2. Meanwhile, in a bowl, mix the remaining ingredients for seasoning.

3. When cooled, peel the eggs and transfer to serving plates. Sprinkle the eggs with some seasoning mixture and serve immediately.

STORAGE: Store this seasoning in the sealed jar in the fridge for up to six months.

SERVE IT WITH: Serve these eggs with avocado slices on the side.

PER SERVING

calories: 230 | fat: 17.2g | total carbs: 6.0g | fiber: 2.0g | protein: 14.9g

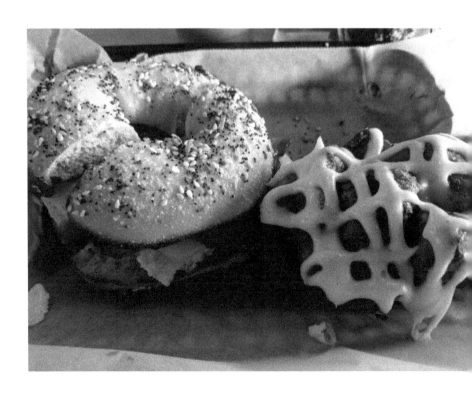

Beef & Veggie Hash

Macros: Fat: 64% | Protein: 27% | Carbs: 9%

Prep time: 15 minutes | Cook time: 35 minutes | Serves 4

One of the best ways to enjoy beef and veggies in your breakfast. This beef and veggie hash alongside eggs give you a healthy choice to start your day.

2 tablespoons olive oil

½ pound (227 g) ground beef

½ of zucchini, chopped

½ of red bell pepper, seeded and chopped

¼ of onion, chopped

2 teaspoons garlic, minced

1½ cups sugar-free tomato sauce

1 tablespoon dried basil, crushed

1 teaspoon dried oregano, crushed

Sea salt and ground black pepper, to taste

4 eggs

1. In a large deep saucepan, heat the oil over medium-high heat and cook the beef for about 10 minutes or until browned, stirring occasionally.

2. Add the zucchini, bell pepper, onion and garlic to cook for about 3 minutes, stirring frequently.

3. Stir in the tomato sauce, dried herbs, salt and black pepper, then bring to a gentle boil. Cook for about 10 minutes, stirring occasionally.

4. With the back of a spoon, make 4 wells in the beef mixture. Carefully, crack 1 egg into each well. Reduce the heat to medium-low and cook covered for about 9 to 10 minutes or until desired doneness.

5. Remove from the heat and serve warm.

STORAGE: Transfer the cooked beef and veggie mixture into a large container and refrigerate for 1 to 2 days.

SERVE IT WITH: Fresh green salad goes great with this dish.

PER SERVING

calories: 268 | fat: 19.2g | total carbs: 8.0g | fiber: 2.0g | protein: 17.8g

Eggs & Spinach Florentine

Macros: Fat: 60% | Protein: 36% | Carbs: 4%

Prep time: 10 minutes | Cook time: 5 minutes | Serves 2

A classic egg Florentine that is perfect for an indulgent breakfast! This classic Eggs Florentine recipe is made with Parmesan spinach with poached eggs.

1 cup fresh spinach leaves, washed completely

2 tablespoons Parmesan cheese, grated freshly

Sea salt and ground black pepper, to taste

1 tablespoon white vinegar

2 eggs

1. In a microwave-safe dish, place the spinach and microwave on High for about 1 to 2 minutes. Remove the bowl from microwave and cut the spinach into bite-sized pieces. Transfer the spinach onto 2 serving plates and sprinkle with Parmesan cheese, salt and black pepper.

2. In a pan of simmering water, add the vinegar and with a spoon, stir quickly. Carefully, break an egg into the center of simmering water. Turn off the heat and cover the pan until the egg is set. Repeat with the remaining egg.

3. Top each plate of spinach with 1 egg and serve.

STORAGE: Transfer the steamed spinach in a container and store in the refrigerator for 1 to 2 days.

REHEAT: Reheat the spinach in microwave and top with poached eggs before serving.

SERVE IT WITH: Serve it with bacon slices.

PER SERVING

calories: 87 | fat: 5.8g | total carbs: 1.1g | fiber: 0.3g | protein: 7.9g

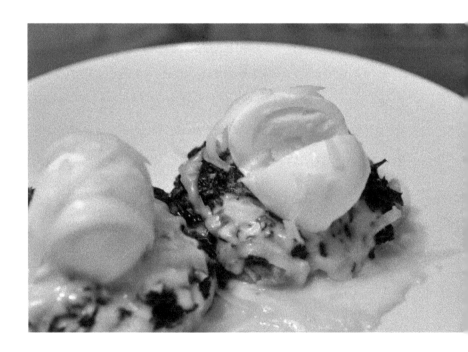

Walnut Granola

Macros: Fat 84% | Protein 11% | Carbs 5%
Prep time: 10 minutes | Cook time: 1 hour | Serves 8

T he nut granola is a versatile meal. The addition of nuts makes it a nutritious keto diet. You can omit or add other ingredients to suit your preference.

1 cup raw sunflower seeds

2 cups shredded coconut, unsweetened

½ cup walnuts

1 cup almonds, sliced

½ cup raw pumpkin seeds

½ teaspoon nutmeg, ground

10 drops liquid stevia

½ cup coconut oil, melted

1 teaspoon cinnamon, ground

1. Preheat the oven to 250°F (120ºC) and line two baking sheets with parchment paper.

2. In a bowl, add the sunflower seeds, shredded coconut, walnuts, almonds, and pumpkin seeds. Toss well to mix.

3. Add the nutmeg, stevia, coconut oil, and cinnamon in a small bowl, and stir thoroughly to blend.

4. Make the granola mixture: Pour the nutmeg mixture into the sunflower seed mixture and blend well to coat the nuts.
5. Spread the granola mixture on the baking sheets. Arrange the sheets in the preheated oven.
6. Bake for 1 hour or until the granola is crispy and lightly browned. Stir the granola every 15 minutes to break the large pieces.
7. Transfer to serving bowls to cool for 8 minutes before serving.

STORAGE: Store in an airtight container in the fridge for up to 4 days or in the freezer for up to 1 month.

REHEAT: Microwave, covered, until it reaches the desired temperature.

SERVE IT WITH: To make this a complete meal, serve with a cup of unsweetened coffee.

PER SERVING

calories: 397 | fat: 37.0g | total carbs: 10.0g | fiber: 5.0g | protein: 11.0g

Creamy Bacon Omelet
Macros: Fat 81% | Protein 15% | Carbs 4%
Prep time: 10 minutes | Cook time: 10 minutes | Serves 4

T he meal is easy to prepare and takes a short time to cook. The bacon and pepper add taste and flavor to the meal. You should definitely try out this recipe.

6 eggs

8 cooked and chopped bacon slices

2 tablespoons heavy whipping cream

1 tablespoon olive oil

¼ cup onion, chopped

½ cup canned artichoke hearts, chopped

Sea salt and ground black pepper, to taste

1. In a bowl, whisk the eggs. Add the bacon and cream, then mix well to blend.

2. Heat the olive oil in a skillet over medium-high heat.

3. Sauté the onion in the skillet for 3 minutes or until tender.

4. Make the omelet: Pour the egg mixture into the skillet and swirl the pan so the mixture covers the bottom evenly.

5. Cook the omelet for about 2 minutes. Lift the edges with a spatula to allow the uncooked egg below spread.

6. Sprinkle the artichoke on the omelet, then flip. Cook for an additional 4 minutes or until the omelet becomes firm. Flip again to keep the artichoke on top. Sprinkle salt and pepper to season.

7. Transfer to serving plates to cool before serving.

STORAGE: Store in an airtight container in the fridge for up to 4 days or in the freezer for up to 1 month.

REHEAT: Microwave, covered, until it reaches the desired temperature.

SERVE IT WITH: To make this a complete meal, serve with a light salad.

PER SERVING

calories: 422 | fat: 38.0g | total carbs: 6.0g | fiber: 2.0g | protein: 16.0g

Sausage Breakfast

Macros: Fat 76% | Protein 22% | Carbs 2%

Prep time: 10 minutes | Cook time: 50 minutes | Serves 8

T he sausage breakfast is filled with a delicious egg mixture over a crescent crust. The meal is easy to prepare and takes a short time to cook.

2 tablespoons olive oil, divided

1 pound (454 g) homemade sausage

8 large eggs

1 tablespoon fresh oregano, chopped

2 cups cooked spaghetti squash

Sea salt and ground black pepper to taste

½ cup Cheddar cheese, shredded

1. Preheat the oven to 375°F (190°C) and grease a casserole dish with 1 tablespoon of olive oil.

2. Heat the remaining olive oil in a skillet. Add the sausages and cook for 5 minutes or until they are browned.

3. In a bowl, break the eggs and whisk well. Add oregano and squash, then mix well. Add salt and pepper to season. Add the sausage, then stir to mix.

4. Pour the sausage mixture in the casserole dish.

5. Scatter the cheese over the mixture and cover loosely with an aluminum foil.
6. Bake in the preheated oven for about 30 minutes. Remove the aluminum foil, then bake for 15 minutes more.
7. Allow the casserole to cool for about 8 minutes before serving.

STORAGE: Store in an airtight container in the fridge for up to 4 days or in the freezer for up to 1 month.

REHEAT: Microwave, covered, until it reaches the desired temperature.

SERVE IT WITH: To make this a complete meal, serve with chocolate peanut butter smoothie.

PER SERVING

calories: 297 | fat: 25.0g | total carbs: 4.0g | fiber: 2.0g | protein: 18.0g

Chicken And Egg Stuffed Avocado

Macros: Fat 71% | Protein 24% | Carbs 5%

Prep time: 10 minutes | Cook time: 20 minutes | Serves 4

A vocado and chicken blend in well in eggs. Salt and pepper add spice to the dish. The meal is perfect for breakfast.

2 peeled and pitted avocados, halved lengthwise

4 eggs

1 (4-ounce / 113-g) cooked chicken breast, shredded

¼ cup Cheddar cheese, shredded

Sea salt and freshly ground black pepper, to taste

1. Preheat the oven to 425°F (220°C).

2. Double the size of the hole in each avocado half with a spoon and arrange on a baking dish, hollow parts facing up.

3. In every hole, crack an egg and divide the chicken breast between every half of the avocado. Sprinkle with the Cheddar cheese and add salt and pepper to season.

4. Bake for about 20 minutes or until the eggs are cooked through.

5. Transfer to four serving plates and serve while warm.

STORAGE: Store in an airtight container in the fridge for up to 4 days or in the freezer for up to 1 month.

REHEAT: Microwave, covered, until it reaches the desired temperature.

SERVE IT WITH: To make this a complete meal, serve with strawberry zucchini chia smoothie.

PER SERVING

calories: 330 | fat: 26.0g | total carbs: 8.0g | fiber: 4.0g | protein: 20.0g

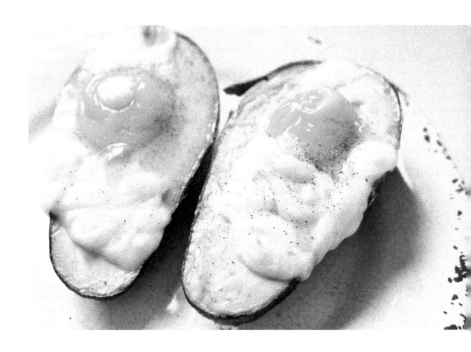

Bacon And Broccoli Egg Muffins
Macros: Fat 66% | Protein 31% | Carbs 3%

Prep time: 20 minutes | Cook time: 15 minutes | Serves 3

The broccoli egg muffins are packed with protein and low net carb which provides a healthy diet. The meal is recommended for breakfast because it sustains your energy for the whole day.

1 cup broccoli, chopped

3 slices bacon

6 beaten eggs

½ teaspoon black pepper, ground

¼ teaspoon garlic powder

½ teaspoon salt

A few drops of Sriracha hot sauce

1 cup Cheddar cheese, shredded

SPECIAL EQUIPMENT:

A 6-cup muffin pan

1. Preheat the oven to 350°F (180°C) and line 6 cups of muffin pan with silicone liners. Set aside.

2. Boil the broccoli in a pot of water for 6 to 8 minutes or until tender, then chop into ¼-inch pieces. Set aside.

3. In a nonstick skillet, fry the slices of bacon for about 8 minutes until crispy, then lay on a paper towel to drain.

4. In a bowl, pour the beaten eggs. Add pepper, garlic, hot sauce, and salt. Whisk well to mix.

5. Put the broccoli into the muffin cups. Top with the bacon, Cheddar cheese, and the egg mixture.

6. Bake in the preheated oven for 25 minutes or until eggs are set.

7. Transfer to serving plates to cool before serving.

STORAGE: Store in an airtight container in the fridge for up to 4 days or in the freezer for up to 1 month.

REHEAT: Microwave, covered, until it reaches the desired temperature.

SERVE IT WITH: To make this a complete meal, serve with coconut blackberry mint smoothie.

PER SERVING

calories: 296 | fat: 21.6g | total carbs: 6.5g | fiber: 4.0g | protein: 23.0g

Scrambled Eggs with Cheese and Chili
Macros: Fat 68% | Protein 29% | Carbs 3%

Prep time: 5 minutes | Cook time: 5 minutes | Serves 2

The scrambled eggs with chili is a magnificent way to start the day, they're packed with flavor and contain nutrients that offer a hearty southern breakfast. The best part is they take a short time to prepare.

4 large eggs

1½ teaspoons butter, unsalted

½ cup warm homemade chili

Salt and ground black pepper, to taste

½ sliced avocado

¼ cup sour cream

¼ cup Cheddar cheese, shredded

1. Whisk the eggs in a bowl.
2. In a skillet, add the butter and heat to melt. Add the eggs then sauté until scrambled. Add the chili, then stir to mix.
3. Add salt and pepper to season.
4. Transfer to serving plates and serve with avocado, sour cream, and cheese.

STORAGE: Store in an airtight container in the fridge for up to 4 days or in the freezer for up to 1 month.

REHEAT: Microwave, covered, until it reaches the desired temperature.

SERVE IT WITH: To make this a complete meal, serve with cinnamon raspberry breakfast smoothie.

PER SERVING

calories: 496| fat: 37.6g | total carbs: 8.2g | fiber: 4.0g | protein: 35.3g

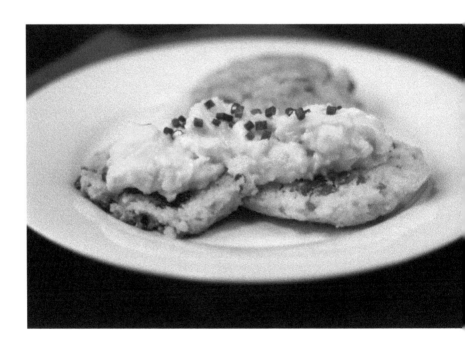

Stevia Chocolate Waffle

Macros: Fat 71% | Protein 23% | Carbs 6%

Prep time: 5 minutes | Cook time: 5 minutes | Serves 1

The stevia chocolate waffle provides the solution for morning carb cravings. The ingredients are easily found on hand and make a fantastic breakfast or brunch option.

1 tablespoon olive oil

⅓ cup almond flour, blanched

½ tablespoon coconut flour

4 drops liquid stevia

2 large eggs, beaten

¼ teaspoon baking powder

¼ teaspoon vanilla extract

1 tablespoon chocolate chips

SPECIAL EQUIPMENT:

A waffle maker

1. Preheat the waffle maker to medium-high heat and grease the waffle maker with olive oil.

2. In a bowl, add the almond flour, coconut flour, stevia, eggs, baking powder, and vanilla. Blend well until it achieves the desired smooth consistency. Fold in the chocolate chips.

3. Pour the mixture into the waffle maker. Cook for about
   5 minutes or until lightly browned.

4. Transfer to serving plates to cool before serving.

STORAGE: Store in an airtight container in the fridge for
up to 4 days or in the freezer for up to 1 month.

REHEAT: Microwave, covered, until it reaches the
desired temperature.

SERVE IT WITH: To make this a complete meal, serve
with plain Greek yogurt.

PER SERVING

calories: 409 | fat: 32.0g | total carbs: 14.0g | fiber: 7.8g
| protein: 24.0g

Almond Cream Cheese Pancakes

Macros: Fat 77% | Protein 18% | Carbs 5%

Prep time: 15 minutes | Cook time: 15 minutes | Serves 1

T he cream cheese pancakes are tender and fluffy, offering a perfect low-carb diet. They are super delicious and extra fluffy.

2 medium eggs

2 ounces (57 g) cream cheese

¼ cup almond flour, blanched

½ teaspoon vanilla extract

¼ teaspoon baking powder

1 teaspoon Swerve

1 tablespoon coconut oil

Salted butter, optional

1. In a blender, break the eggs and add cheese, almond flour, vanilla, baking powder, and Swerve. Process until the mixture is smooth and foamy.

2. Make the pancakes: Grease a skillet with coconut oil and heat. Drop one-third of the batter into the skillet and cook for 6 minutes. Flip the pancake halfway through the cooking time. Repeat with the remaining batter.

3. Transfer to serving plates and top with the salted butter, if desired.

STORAGE: Store in an airtight container in the fridge for up to 4 days or in the freezer for up to 1 month.

REHEAT: Microwave, covered, until it reaches the desired temperature.

SERVE IT WITH: To make this a complete meal, serve with pumpkin spice smoothie.

PER SERVING

calories: 481 | fat: 41.0g | total carbs: 12.0g | fiber: 6.0g | protein: 22.0g

Simple Scrambled Eggs

Macros: Fat 68% | Protein 31% | Carbs 1%

Prep time: 10 minutes | Cook time: 15 minutes | Serves 2

S crambled eggs provide a scrumptious breakfast option. The scrambled eggs are easy to prepare and take a short time to cook.

1 tablespoon unsalted butter

1 cup white mushrooms, sliced

4 large scrambled eggs

⅓ cup crumbled goat cheese

2 fresh chopped basil leaves

⅓ cup chopped bacon, cooked

Salt and freshly ground black pepper, to taste

1. In a skillet, add the butter and heat to melt. Add the mushrooms and sauté for about 5 minutes or until soft.
2. Break the eggs in the skillet and sauté for about 5 minutes or until scrambled.
3. Add the cheese, basil, and bacon over the mushroom mixture and sauté for 2 minutes or until the cheese melts. Add salt and pepper to season.
4. Transfer to serving plates and serve warm.

STORAGE: Store in an airtight container in the fridge for up to 4 days or in the freezer for up to 1 month.

REHEAT: Microwave, covered, until it reaches the desired temperature.

SERVE IT WITH: To make this a complete meal, serve with sautéed spinach on the side.

PER SERVING

calories: 384 | fat: 29.0g | total carbs: 3.0g | fiber: 1.6g | protein: 29.4g

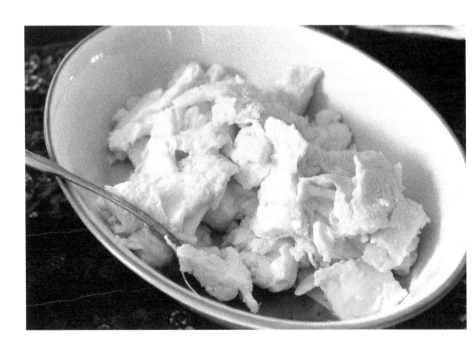

Basic Capicola Egg Cups

Macros: Fat 74% | Protein 23% | Carbs 3%

Prep time: 5 minutes | Cook time: 14 minutes | Serves 3

C apicola egg cups offer a variety as far as eggs go. They are super delicious and ensures an excellent breakfast to kick-start your day. Prepare the egg cups easily and in a brief period.

1 tablespoon olive oil

6 slices capicola

¾ cup Cheddar cheese, shredded

6 large eggs

Salt and freshly ground black pepper, to taste

Thinly sliced basil, for garnish

SPECIAL EQUIPMENT:

A 6-cup muffin pan

1. Preheat the oven to 400°F (205°C) and grease the muffin cups with olive oil.

2. Put each slice of the capicola into each cup to form a bowl shape.

3. Sprinkle 2 tablespoons of cheese into every cup.

4. In every cup, crack an egg, then add salt and pepper to season.

5. Bake for about 14 minutes, or until eggs are set.

6. Garnish with the basil, then serve warm.

STORAGE: Store in an airtight container in the fridge for up to 4 days or in the freezer for up to 1 month.

REHEAT: Microwave, covered, until it reaches the desired temperature.

SERVE IT WITH: To make this a complete meal, serve with keto green lemon smoothie.

PER SERVING

calories: 307 | fat: 25.3g | total carbs: 2.3g | fiber: 0g | protein: 17.4g

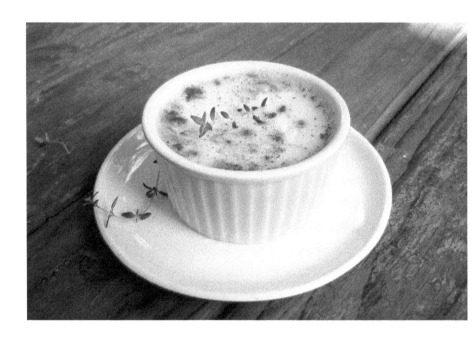

Easy Sausage, Egg, And Cheese Casserole
Macros: Fat 81% | Protein 17% | Carbs 2%

Prep time: 15 minutes | Cook time: 35 minutes | Serves 4

H ere's a scrumptious breakfast casserole that the entire family will love. The meal is quick and easy to prepare for a crowd. Bacon can also be used in place of sausage according to your preference.

2 tablespoons coconut oil

1 tablespoon butter, unsalted

⅓ cup yellow onions, chopped

1 pound (454 g) bulk breakfast sausage

6 whisked eggs

1 pressed clove garlic

⅓ cup heavy whipping cream

½ teaspoon ground black pepper

1 teaspoon salt

1 cup Cheddar cheese, shredded

1. Preheat the oven to 350°F (180°C) and coat a baking dish lightly with coconut oil.

2. In a skillet, add the butter and heat to melt. Add the onions then sauté for about 4 minutes until soft.

3. Add the sausage, then cook for about 5 minutes until browned evenly. Drain excess butter and set aside until ready to use.

4. In a bowl, add the whisked eggs, garlic, cream, pepper, and salt, then whisk together thoroughly.

5. Evenly spread the sausage on the baking dish, then top with cheese. Add the egg mixture.

6. Bake for about 35 minutes until the edges begin to brown.

7. Transfer to serving plates to cool for about 5 minutes before serving.

STORAGE: Store in an airtight container in the fridge for up to 4 days or in the freezer for up to 1 month.

REHEAT: Microwave, covered, until it reaches the desired temperature.

SERVE IT WITH: To make this a complete meal, serve it with a cup of unsweetened coconut milk.

PER SERVING

calories: 977 | fat: 88.2g | total carbs: 5.0g | fiber: 0.2g | protein: 41.1g

Waffle Sandwiches

Macros: Fat 78% | Protein 18% | Carbs 5%

Prep time: 10 minutes | Cook time: 20 minutes | Serves 2

T his is a wonderful combination for a breakfast sandwich that is savory. You can play around by swapping the waffle sandwich ingredients, like going for ham instead of bacon!

WAFFLES:

2 large eggs, whisked

¼ teaspoon baking powder

½ tablespoon coconut flour

⅓ cup almond flour, blanched

Pinch of salt

4 drops liquid stevia

¼ teaspoon vanilla extract

SANDWICH FILLING:

4 slices bacon

2 eggs

2 slices Cheddar cheese, shredded

½ sliced avocado

Salt and ground black pepper, to taste

SPECIAL EQUIPMENT:

A waffle maker

1. Preheat a waffle maker to medium-high heat.
2. Make the waffles: In a mixing bowl, add the whisked eggs, baking powder, coconut flour, almond flour, salt, stevia, and vanilla and whisk well until smooth.
3. Transfer the batter into the waffle maker and cook for about 5 minutes until golden brown and a little crisp.
4. Meantime, make the sandwich filling: In a nonstick skillet, fry the bacon over medium-high heat for 8 minutes until crispy. Remove the bacon from the skillet and leave the bacon grease in the skillet.
5. Crack the eggs in the skillet, and cook to make the yolks runny.
6. Flip the eggs, then top each egg with a slice of the Cheddar cheese. Cover the skillet to allow the cheese to melt.
7. Make the sandwich: Quarter the waffle with a knife. Lay the quarters on two serving plates, then top each waffle with 2 bacon slices and the egg with cheese toppings, finished by avocado slices. Add salt and pepper to season.
8. Top each sandwich with the remaining quarters and serve.

STORAGE: Store in an airtight container in the fridge for up to 4 days or in the freezer for up to 1 month.

REHEAT: Microwave, covered, until it reaches the desired temperature.

SERVE IT WITH: To make this a complete meal, serve with keto coffee.

PER SERVING calories: 666 | fat: 57.9g | total carbs: 10.7g | fiber: 3.4g | protein: 28.9g

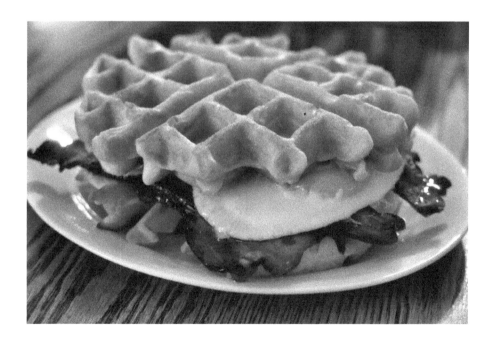

Lemon Allspice Muffins

Macros: Fat 84% | Protein 13% | Carbs 3%

Prep time: 15 minutes | Cook time: 25 minutes | Serves 12

A llspice muffins are a delicious buttery, crumbly and sweet treat. The muffins are light and tender and get a kick from the allspice batter. The simplicity of the recipe and process produces delicious results.

1½ cups almond flour, blanched

½ cup flaxseeds, roughly ground

½ cup erythritol

2 teaspoons baking powder

1 tablespoon plus 1 teaspoon ground allspice

½ teaspoon ground gray sea salt

6 large whisked eggs

½ cup unsweetened coconut milk

½ cup melted coconut oil

1 teaspoon vanilla extract

Grated zest 1 lemon

TOPPING:

¼ cup walnut pieces, raw

SPECIAL EQUIPMENT:

A 12-cup muffin pan

1. Preheat the oven to 350°F (180°C) and line a muffin pan with 12 paper liners. Set aside.
2. In a bowl, add the almond flour, flaxseeds, erythritol, baking powder, allspice, and salt, then mix to blend.
3. In another bowl, add the eggs, coconut milk, coconut oil, vanilla, and lemon zest, then mix well. Add the almond flour mixture, then stir well with a spatula.
4. Divide the batter into the muffin cups, then sprinkle the walnuts on top.
5. Bake in the preheated oven until the top becomes golden for about 25 minutes.
6. Transfer to a wire rack to cool for about 10 minutes before serving.

STORAGE: Store in an airtight container in the refrigerator for up to 4 days or in the freezer for up to 1 month.

REHEAT: Microwave, covered, until it reaches the desired temperature.

SERVE IT WITH: To make this a complete meal, serve with perfect keto Frappuccino.

PER SERVING

calories: 260 | fat: 24.2g | total carbs: 5.8g | fiber: 3.4g | protein: 8.2g

Keto Cinnamon Flaxseed Bun Muffins

Macros: Fat 86% | Protein 11% | Carbs 3%

Prep time: 10 minutes | Cook time: 15 minutes | Serves 12

T he keto cinnamon buns are a marvellous way to start your day. Naturally high in fiber, low in carbohydrates, sugar-free and paleo-friendly. They are gluten-free, dairy-free and sugar-free, hence provide a healthier option.

2 cups flaxseeds, roughly ground

2 tablespoons ground cinnamon

⅓ cup erythritol

½ teaspoon gray sea salt, finely ground

1 tablespoon baking powder

5 large whisked eggs

⅓ cup melted coconut oil

½ cup water

¼ teaspoon liquid stevia

2 teaspoons vanilla extract

SPECIAL EQUIPMENT:

A 12-cup muffin pan

1. Preheat the oven to 350°F (180°C) and line a muffin pan with 12 paper liners. Set aside.

2. In a bowl, add the flaxseeds, cinnamon, erythritol, salt, and baking powder, then stir to combine.
3. Add the eggs, oil, water, stevia, and vanilla in a blender, then pulse until bubbly.
4. Pour the egg mixture into the flaxseed mixture and stir with a spatula until the batter becomes very fluffy. Allow the batter to sit for about 3 minutes.
5. Divide the batter into the muffin cups. Bake in the preheated oven for about 15 minutes.
6. Remove the pan from the oven to a wire rack to cool for about 20 minutes before serving.

STORAGE: Store in an airtight container in the fridge for up to 4 days or in the freezer for up to 1 month.

REHEAT: Microwave, covered, until it reaches the desired temperature.

SERVE IT WITH: To make this a complete meal, serve with sugar-free chocolate sea salt smoothies.

PER SERVING

calories: 254 | fat: 24.2g | total carbs: 8.8g | fiber: 6.4g | protein: 6.7g

Bacon Quiche

Macros: Fat 71% | Protein 24% | Carbs 5%

Prep time: 20 minutes | Cook time: 50 minutes | Serves 8

T he bacon quiche can be prepared ahead of time. They are highly recommended for breakfast. The bacon quiche will definitely become a family favorite. Ingredients can be adjusted to your liking.

CRUST:

2 tablespoons melted lard, plus more for greasing the tart pans

2 cups almond flour, blanched

1 large egg

⅛ teaspoon gray sea salt, finely ground

FILLING:

6 strips (6-ounce / 170-g) bacon

1⅓ cups unsweetened coconut milk

¼ cup plus 2 tablespoons nutritional yeast

4 large beaten eggs

⅛ teaspoon ground nutmeg

¼ teaspoon ground black pepper

¼ teaspoon gray sea salt, finely ground

1. Preheat the oven to 350°F (180°C) and lightly grease the tart pans with melted lard. Set aside.

2. Make the crusts: In a bowl, add the almond flour, lard, egg, and salt and whisk well to form a dough.

3. Divide the dough into 4 pieces, then lay each piece in the tart pan. Use a rounded spatula to press the dough into ⅛ inch.

4. Lay the tart pans on the baking sheet and bake in the preheated oven until the crusts become lightly golden for about 15 minutes.

5. Make the filling: In a frying pan, add the bacon and cook over medium-high heat until crispy. Remove from the pan, then roughly chop the bacon.

6. In another bowl, add coconut milk, yeast, eggs, nutmeg, pepper, and salt. Add the bacon then whisk well to combine.

7. Remove the crusts from oven and adjust the temperature to 325°F (160°C). Fill the crusts evenly with the filling.

8. Return the crusts to the oven. Bake for about 30 minutes until the tops turn lightly golden.

9. Transfer to a wire rack to cool before serving.

STORAGE: Store in an airtight container in the fridge for up to 4 days or in the freezer for up to 1 month.

REHEAT: Microwave, covered, until it reaches the desired temperature.

SERVE IT WITH: To make this a complete meal, serve with keto collagen smoothie.

PER SERVING

calories: 387 | fat: 30.6g | total carbs: 11.0g | fiber: 6.0g | protein: 22.8g

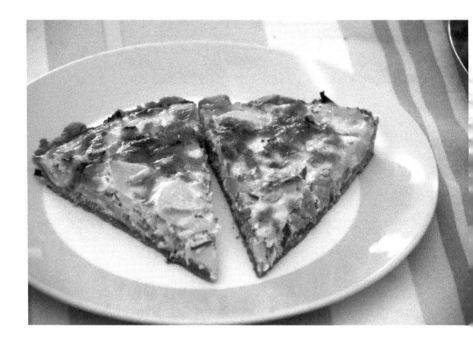

Low Carb Jambalaya with Chicken
Macros: Fat 76% | Protein 20% | Carbs 4%

Prep time: 25 minutes | Cook time: 25 minutes | Serves 4

J ambalaya is easy to make and allows you to experiment with your favorite protein. The meal is full of tasty flavors that brings everyone together.

⅓ cup lard

4 (8-ounce / 227-g) cooked and chopped sausage

1 cup cubed skinless chicken thighs, cooked

½ cup green onions, chopped

1¼ cups diced celery

2 tablespoons Cajun seasoning

½ cup chicken broth

2½ cups riced cauliflower

¼ cup diced tomatoes

Handful of freshly chopped parsley

1. In a frying pan, add the lard and heat to melt. Add the sausage, chicken thighs, green onions, celery, and Cajun seasoning. Cook for about 10 minutes until the celery softens, stirring occasionally.

2. Add the chicken broth and riced cauliflower. Cover and cook for about 5 minutes until the cauliflower is tender.

3. Add the diced tomatoes and stir. Increase the heat and cook uncovered for about 7 minutes, or until the liquid has evaporated.

4. Remove from heat to four bowls, then top with the parsley. Allow to cool for 5 minutes before serving.

STORAGE: Store in an airtight container in the fridge for up to 4 days.

REHEAT: Microwave, covered, until it reaches the desired temperature.

SERVE IT WITH: To make this a complete meal, serve with slow-cooked mushroom and chicken soup.

PER SERVING

calories: 446 | fat: 37.7g | total carbs: 7.6g | fiber: 3.4g | protein: 22.5g

Sausage And Spinach Hash Bowl

Macros: Fat 84% | Protein 12% | Carbs 4%

Prep time: 25 minutes | Cook time: 25 minutes |Serves 2

S ausage and spinach hash bowl offers a satisfying and scrumptious brunch that will keep you going throughout the day. It is fast to cook and good for your health because of all the vegetables ingredients.

HASH:

⅔ cup peeled radishes, cut into ½-inch cubes

2 tablespoons lard

¼ cup green onions, chopped (green parts only)

2 (4-ounce / 113-g) precooked sausages, cut into ½-inch cubes

FOR THE BOWLS:

2 cups fresh spinach

½ large sliced Hass avocado

2 cooked bacon, chopped into ½-inch strips

1 teaspoon fresh parsley, chopped

1. Steam the radishes until tender for about 10 minutes.

2. Make the hash: In a frying pan over medium-high heat, add the lard and heat to melt. Add the radishes then cook until the radishes turn brown, about 10 minutes.

3. Add the green onions and sausages then cook until the sausages turn brown, about 5 minutes.
4. Assemble the bowls: Equally divide the spinach into 2 serving bowls. Once the hash cooked through, divide between the bowls equally, laying them on top of the spinach bed.
5. Top with equal amounts of the avocado, bacon, and parsley before serving.

STORAGE: Store in an airtight container in the fridge for up to 4 days.

REHEAT: Microwave, covered, until it reaches the desired temperature.

SERVE IT WITH: To make this a complete meal, serve with vanilla milkshake.

PER SERVING

calories: 536 | fat: 49.8g | total carbs: 10.4g | fiber: 5.0g | protein: 16.5g

Healthy Hemp Seed Porridge

Macros: Fat 82% | Protein 16% | Carbs 2%

Prep time: 2 minutes | Cook time: 5 minutes | Serves 2

M ade with seeds, nuts, vanilla extract and cinnamon, hemp seed porridge is keto-friendly. Taste very similar to oatmeal but is low in carbs and high in protein and fat. Takes a very short time to prepare.

PORRIDGE:

1 cup unsweetened almond milk

½ cup hemp seeds, hulled

1 tablespoon chia seeds

2 tablespoons flaxseeds, roughly ground

2 tablespoons coconut oil

1 tablespoon erythritol

¾ teaspoon vanilla extract

¾ teaspoon ground cinnamon

¼ cup almond meal

TOPPINGS:

4 raw Brazil nuts, roughly chopped

2 tablespoons hemp seeds, hulled

Fresh berries, optional

1. In a saucepan, add the milk, hemp seeds, chia seeds, flaxseeds, coconut oil, erythritol, vanilla, and

cinnamon. Stir well to combine. Heat over medium-high heat and bring to a boil.

2. As it bubbles, stir well and cover. Cook for about 2 minutes.

3. Remove the mixture from the heat, then add almond meal and stir. Divide equally between 2 bowls. Top each of bowls equally with the Brazil nuts, hemp seeds, and berries before serving.

STORAGE: Store in an airtight container in the fridge for up to 4 days or in the freezer for up to 1 month.

REHEAT: Microwave, covered, until it reaches the desired temperature.

SERVE IT WITH: To make this a complete meal, serve with low-carb strawberry smoothie.

PER SERVING

calories: 610 | fat: 55.6g | total carbs: 15.2g | fiber: 12.4g | protein: 24.6g

Nut-Free Granola with Clusters

Macros: Fat 79% | Protein 17% | Carbs 4%

Prep time: 20 minutes | Cook time: 50 minutes | Serves 12

T he granola recipe is nut-free but is rich with a burst of flavor. The crunchy granola is simple and easy to make and is ready for the oven in a short time. Nut-free granola provides an excellent alternative for people allergic to nuts.

GRANOLA:

½ cup melted coconut oil, plus more for greasing the pan

1 large whisked egg

½ cup collagen peptides

3 tablespoons ground cinnamon

¼ teaspoon liquid stevia

2 teaspoons vanilla extract

¼ teaspoon finely ground gray sea salt

2 cups shredded coconut, unsweetened

1 cup hemp seeds, hulled

¼ cup chia seeds

1 cup sesame seeds

TOPPING:

Unsweetened coconut milk, as needed

Fresh berries, as needed

1. Preheat the oven to 300°F (150°C) and grease a baking pan with coconut oil. Set aside.
2. Make the granola: In a bowl, pour the egg, coconut oil, collagen, cinnamon, stevia, vanilla, and salt and whisk to combine.
3. In another bowl, add the shredded coconut, hemp seeds, chia seeds, and sesame seeds and mix well. Pour in the egg mixture and stir using a spatula to coat all the seeds.
4. Transfer to the greased baking pan and firmly press the mixture down with a spatula.
5. Bake for about 30 minutes until the corners and top start to turn golden.
6. Using a spatula to split granola into pieces. Flip them over, then bake for 20 minutes more until they turn golden.
7. Let the clusters cool for about 30 minutes. Transfer to serving bowls and pour in the coconut milk. Top with the berries and serve.

STORAGE: Store in an airtight container in the fridge for up to 4 days or in the freezer for up to 1 month.

REHEAT: Microwave, covered, until it reaches the desired temperature.

SERVE IT WITH: To make this a complete meal, serve with minty green protein smoothie.

PER SERVING

calories: 351 | fat: 31.0g | total carbs: 9.9g | fiber: 6.4g | protein: 14.5g

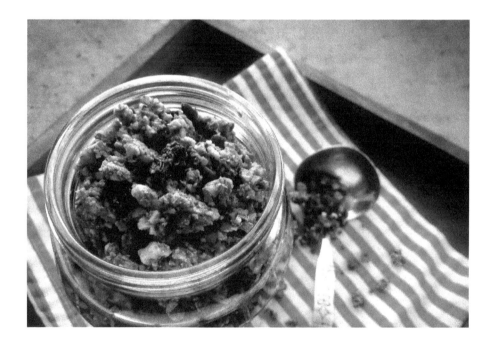

Creamy Spanish Scrambled Eggs

Macros: Fat 85% | Protein 10% | Carbs 5%

Prep time: 10 minutes | Cook time: 10 minutes | Serves 2

S panish scramble is the best scrambled eggs that can easily be prepared for breakfast. Pepper is added to spice it up.

¼ cup heavy whipping cream

2 tablespoons finely chopped cilantro

4 large whisked eggs

Salt and black pepper, to taste

3 tablespoons butter

1 Serrano chili pepper

1 small chopped tomato

2 tablespoons sliced scallions

1. In a bowl, add the cream, cilantro, eggs, pepper, and salt and mix well.
2. In a pan, add the butter and heat to melt. Mix in Serrano pepper and tomatoes then sauté for 2 minutes over medium heat. Add cream mixture to the pan and sauté for 4 minutes or until scrambled.
3. Top with the scallions for garnish before serving.

STORAGE: Store in an airtight container in the fridge for up to 4 days or in the freezer for up to 1 month.

REHEAT: Microwave, covered, until it reaches the desired temperature.

SERVE IT WITH: To make this a complete meal, serve with mocha keto coffee shake.

PER SERVING

calories: 278 | fat: 26.3g | total carbs: 4.1g | fiber: 0.8g | protein: 7.0g

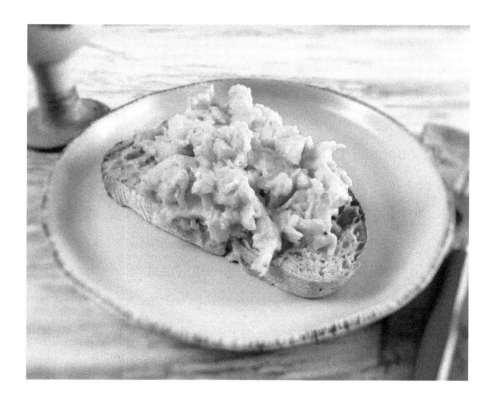

Spanish Egg Frittata

Macros: Fat 86% | Protein 12% | Carbs 2%

Prep time: 6 minutes | Cook time: 40 minutes | Serves 2

T he effort required in making frittata is similar to scrambled eggs. The dish provides an appropriate choice for brunch. Quantity of ingredients can be altered depending on the number of people you're serving.

1 tablespoon olive oil

½ tablespoon butter

1½ ounces (42 g) bacon

2 ounces (57 g) fresh spinach

2 whisked eggs

¼ cup heavy whipped cream

1½ ounces (42 g) shredded Cheddar cheese

Salt and freshly ground black pepper, to taste

1. Preheat the oven to 375°F (190°C) and grease a baking dish with olive oil. Set aside.

2. In a skillet, add the butter and heat to melt, then add the bacon. Cook the bacon until crispy, about 8 minutes. Add the spinach and cook until tender. Remove from the heat to a large bowl.

3. Add the eggs, cream, cheese, salt and pepper into the large bowl, then stir to combine. Transfer the mixture to the baking dish.
4. Bake in the preheated oven for 30 minutes. Cut a small slit in the center, if raw eggs run into the cut, baking for another few minutes.
5. Transfer to serving plates to cool before serving.

STORAGE: Store in an airtight container in the fridge for up to 4 days or in the freezer for up to 1 month.

REHEAT: Microwave, covered, until it reaches the desired temperature.

SERVE IT WITH: To make this a complete meal, serve with strawberry avocado keto smoothie.

PER SERVING

calories: 643 | fat: 61.7g | total carbs: 2.9g | sugars: 0.6g | protein: 19.7g

Basic Cream Crepes
Macros: Fat 82% | Protein 11% | Carbs 7%

Prep time: 5 minutes | Cook time: 20 minutes | Serves 2

T his is an exquisite breakfast with a very rich nutrient content. The dish is simple and easy to prepare. Cream crepes is also appropriate for a low-carb diet.

2 tablespoons melted coconut oil, divided

2 whisked eggs

Sea salt, to taste

1 teaspoon Swerve

2 tablespoons coconut flour

½ cup heavy whipping cream

1. In a bowl, add 1 tablespoon coconut oil, eggs, salt, and Swerve, then whisk to mix.

2. Slowly mix in the coconut flour, then fold in the cream until the mixture is smooth.

3. Heat the remaining oil in a skillet over medium heat. Pout half of the mixture into the skillet. Cook for 2 minutes on each side and repeat the process with the remaining mixture.

4. Transfer to serving plates and serve while warm.

STORAGE: Store in an airtight container in the fridge for up to 4 days or in the freezer for up to 1 month.

REHEAT: Microwave, covered, until it reaches the desired temperature.

SERVE IT WITH: To make this a complete meal, serve with keto cinnamon smoothie.

PER SERVING

calories: 390 | fat: 35.3g | total carbs: 7.4g | fiber: 0g | protein: 10.6g

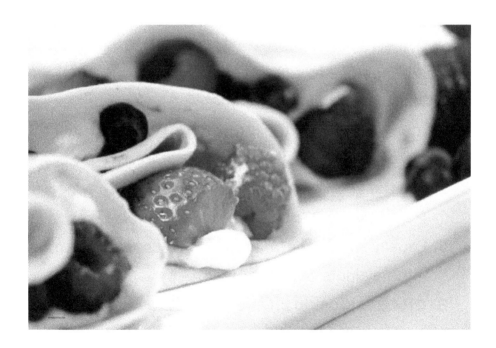

Strawberry Smoothie Bowl

Macros: Fat 58% | Protein 30% | Carbs 12%

Prep time: 15 minutes | Cook time: 0 minutes | Serves 2

T he smoothie bowl is a simple and easy to treat. It requires few ingredients and can be prepared for breakfast or as a snack. Toppings of your choice can also be added.

1 cup frozen strawberries

½ cup plain Greek yogurt

¼ cup almond milk, unsweetened

½ tablespoon whey protein powder, unsweetened

1 tablespoon chopped walnuts

1. In a blender, add the strawberries. Process until it has a smooth consistency.

2. Add the yogurt, almond milk, and protein powder, then process for 2 minutes more to combine well.

3. Equally divide the mixture into 2 bowls, and top with the walnuts before serving.

STORAGE: Store in an airtight container in the fridge for up to 4 days or in the freezer for up to 1 month.

SERVE IT WITH: To make this a complete meal, serve with healthy keto green smoothie.

PER SERVING

calories: 140 | fat: 9.0g | total carbs: 6.0g | fiber: 1.8g | protein: 10.5g

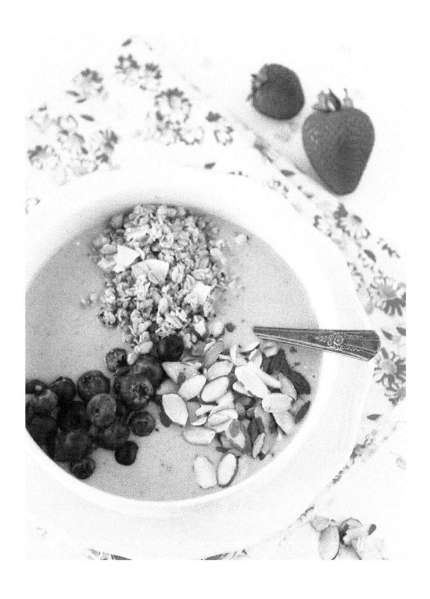

Breadless Egg Sandwich

Macros: Fat 79% | Protein 19% | Carbs 2%

Prep time: 5 minutes | Cook time:16 minutes | Serves 2

W e can try to use our imagination to create more ways of making a gluten-free or 'bread-free' sandwich or other keto-friendly breakfast. Making something wrapped in something have many possibilities to find.

4 slices bacon

2 eggs

Salt and freshly ground black pepper, to taste

⅓ cup Cheddar cheese, shredded

1. Cook the bacon in a nonstick skillet over medium-high heat for 3 to 4 minutes. When it buckles and curls, loosen and flip the bacon slices so they brown evenly and cook for 3 to 4 minutes more.

2. Turn off the heat and crumble the bacon into pieces with a spatula. Transfer to a plate lined with paper towels. Set aside. Leave the bacon grease in the skillet.

3. Gently crack the eggs into the skillet, and sprinkle with salt and pepper.

4. Cook the eggs for 3 minutes until the egg whites are firm. Flip and scatter the eggs with bacon pieces and

shredded cheese, then cook for 3 minutes more until the cheese melts.

5. Remove the eggs from the skillet and serve warm.

STORAGE: Store in an airtight container in the fridge for up to 2 days or keep in the freezer for up to 1 month.

REHEAT: Microwave, covered, until the desired temperature is reached or reheat in a frying pan or air fryer / instant pot, covered, on medium.

SERVE IT WITH: To make this a complete meal, you can serve it with plain Greek yogurt for an enjoyable morning.

PER SERVING

calories: 426 | fat: 37.4g | total carbs: 1.7g | fiber: 0g | protein: 20.7g

Ham And Veggie Omelet in A Bag

Macros: Fat 67% | Protein 28% | Carbs 5%

Prep time: 15 minutes | Cook time:13 minutes | Serves 1

T his recipe shows us a unique way to make an omelet. But I believe the significance of this recipe is far more than an omelet, because it shows us a creative way of making food.

2 eggs

2 slices ham, chopped

1 tablespoon green bell pepper, chopped

2 tablespoons fresh tomato, chopped

2 fresh mushrooms, sliced

1 tablespoon onion, chopped

½ cup Cheddar cheese, shredded

1 tablespoon salsa

1. Whisk the eggs in a bowl, then add the whisked eggs, ham, green bell pepper, tomato, mushroom, onion, cheese, and salsa into a Ziploc bag. Shake the bag to combine well. You can prepare 4 more omelet bags at a time.

2. Bring a pot of water to a boil. Squeeze the air out of the bag and seal. Place the bag into the boiling water and cook for 13 minutes.

3. Remove the bag from the water. Open the bag and serve the omelet on a platter.

STORAGE: Keep in the fridge for up to 3 to 4 days, or wrap in plastic and keep in the fridge for up to 4 weeks.

REHEAT: Microwave, covered, until the desired temperature is reached or reheat in a frying pan or air fryer / instant pot, covered, on medium.

SERVE IT WITH: To make this a complete meal, serve it with something crispy such as avocado sticks.

PER SERVING

calories: 625 | fat: 46.6g | total carbs: 9.3g | fiber: 2.2g | protein: 44.4g

Classic Omelet

Macros: Fat 73% | Protein 22% | Carbs 5%

Prep time: 10 minutes | Cook time: 30 minutes | Serves 6

C lassic is just an example. We can inject it with our own preference and make it become our own 'classic'. The soft and creamy texture will enlighten your appetite and give you an excellent mood for a delightful working day.

9 eggs

½ cup unsweetened coconut milk

½ cup sour cream

1 teaspoon salt

2 green onions, chopped

1 teaspoon butter, melted

¼ cup Cheddar cheese, shredded

1. Start by preheating the oven to 350°F (180°C).
2. Whisk together the eggs, coconut milk, sour cream, and salt in a bowl, then fold in the green onions.
3. Coat a baking pan with the melted butter and tilt the pan so the butter covers the bottom evenly. Pour the egg mixture in the pan.
4. Arrange the pan in the preheated oven and bake for 25 minutes. You can check the doneness by cutting a slit in the center of the frittata, if raw eggs run into

the cut, then baking for another few minutes. Sprinkle with the cheese and continue baking for an additional 2 minutes until the cheese melts.

5. Remove the omelet from the oven and serve warm.

STORAGE: Keep in the fridge for up to 3 to 4 days, or wrap in plastic and keep in the fridge for up to 4 weeks.

REHEAT: Microwave, covered, until the desired temperature is reached or reheat in a frying pan or air fryer / instant pot, covered, on medium.

SERVE IT WITH: To make this a complete meal, serve it with something crispy such as avocado sticks.

PER SERVING

calories: 287 | fat: 23.1g | total carbs: 4.3g | fiber: 0.5g | protein: 15.9g

Paleo Omelet Muffins

Macros: Fat 61% | Protein 31% | Carbs 8%

Prep time: 15 minutes | Cook time: 20 minutes | Serves 4

S mall, cute, and easy made muffins. Its golden color will bring you dynamic to the keto diet. It's just like a little egg flower which holds the bacon up and raises your value on judging a good recipe.

8 eggs

8 ounces (227 g) cooked ham, crumbled

1 cup red bell pepper, diced

1 cup onion, diced

¼ teaspoon salt

⅛ teaspoon ground black pepper

2 tablespoons water

SPECIAL EQUIPMENT:

An 8-cup muffin pan, greased with olive oil

1. Start by preheating the oven to 350ºF (180ºC).
2. Whisk together the eggs, ham, red bell pepper, onion, salt, ground black pepper, and water in a large bowl.
3. Gently pour the mixture into the muffin cups, then arrange the cups in the preheated oven.
4. Bake for 18 minutes or until the tops of muffins spring back when lightly touched with your finger.

5. Remove from the oven. Let stand for a few minutes before serving.

STORAGE: Store in an airtight container for 1 to 2 days or keep in the fridge for up to 1 week.

REHEAT: Microwave, covered, until the desired temperature is reached or reheat in a frying pan or air fryer / instant pot, covered, on medium.

SERVE IT WITH: To make this a complete meal, serve it with a dollop of plain Greek yogurt or other drinks you like.

PER SERVING

calories: 357 | fat: 24.3g | total carbs: 8.3g | fiber: 1.7g | protein: 27.9g

Easy Enchilada Chicken Dip

Macros: Fat 82% | Protein 15% | Carbs 3%

Prep time: 15 minutes | Cook time: 50 minutes | Serves 30

I f you are looking for an amazing appetizer to please your crowd, this Enchilada chicken dip is a solid choice. It's delicious and super easy to prepare. It's perfect when served with some baked keto vegetable chips or raw veggies.

1 pound (454 g) chicken breasts, skin and bones removed

1 (8-ounce / 227-g) jar mayonnaise, keto-friendly

1 (8-ounce / 227-g) package cream cheese, softened

1 (4-ounce / 114-g) can diced red chile peppers

1 (8-ounce / 227-g) package shredded Cheddar cheese

1 jalapeño pepper, diced finely

1. Preheat your oven to 350°F (180°C). Line a baking sheet with parchment paper and set aside.

2. Place the chicken on the prepared baking sheet. Bake for 20 minutes or until the chicken is cooked through.

3. Remove from the oven and let the chicken cool, then shed it using forks on a clean work surface.

4. Transfer the shredded chicken to a medium mixing bowl and add the remaining ingredients. Stir to combine well.
5. Arrange the chicken mixture on the baking sheet and bake uncovered for 30 minutes, or until the edges are browned.
6. Remove from the oven and let it cool for 5 minutes to serve.

STORAGE: Store in an airtight container in the fridge for up to 3 days.

REHEAT: Microwave, covered, until it reaches the desired temperature.

SERVE IT WITH: To make this a delicious and complete meal, serve the dip with some baked keto vegetables or raw veggies.

PER SERVING

calories: 113 | fat: 10.6g | total carbs: 0.9g | fiber: 0.1g | protein: 3.9g

Grilled Portobello Mushrooms
Macros: Fat 80% | Protein 3% | Carbs 17%
Prep time: 10 minutes | Cook time: 10 minutes | Serves 3

T his is a delicious snack food that you can easily make on your grill. Everybody in your family or friends coming over will rave on about how wonderful it is. It's also insanely irresistible, so you will want to make it repeatedly.

3 portobello mushrooms

¼ cup olive oil

4 tablespoons balsamic vinegar

4 garlic cloves, minced

3 tablespoons onions, chopped

1. Thoroughly clean the mushrooms and cut off the stems on your cutting board. Reserve the stems for other use.

2. Place the mushroom caps on a platter, grills facing up. Set aside.

3. Mix the oil, vinegar, garlic, and onions in a small bowl, then pour the mixture evenly over the mushroom caps. Let them rest in the marinade for about 1 hour.

4. Preheat the grill to medium-high heat.

5. Grill the mushrooms for 10 minutes, flipping them halfway through, or until the mushrooms are lightly browned.
6. Transfer to a plate and let cool for 5 minutes before serving.

STORAGE: Store in an airtight container in the fridge for up to 3 days.

REHEAT: Microwave, covered, until it reaches the desired temperature.

SERVE IT WITH: To make this a delicious complete meal, serve the grilled mushrooms with a hearty topping.

PER SERVING

calories: 206 | fat: 18.3g | total carbs: 9.1g | fiber: 1.3g | protein: 2.2g

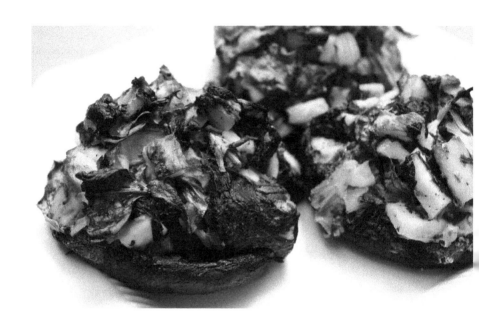

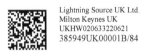

Lightning Source UK Ltd.
Milton Keynes UK
UKHW020633220621
385949UK00001B/84

9 781803 176185